Terry Fox

Terry Barber

MAPLE LEAF
SERIES

Terry Fox is published by
Grass Roots Press, a division of Literacy Services of Canada Ltd.

PHONE 1–888–303–3213
WEBSITE www.grassrootsbooks.net

ACKNOWLEDGMENTS

We acknowledge the financial support of the Government of Canada through
the Canada Book Fund (CBF) for our publishing activities.

Produced with the assistance of
the Government of Alberta, Alberta   **Government**
Multimedia Development Fund.   **of Alberta ■**

Editor: Dr. Pat Campbell
Image research: Terry Fox Foundation and Dr. Pat Campbell
Book design: Lara Minja

Library and Archives Canada Cataloguing in Publication

Barber, Terry, date
    Terry Fox / Terry Barber.

(Maple leaf series)
ISBN 978–1–926583–38–9

1. Fox, Terry, 1958–1981. 2. Cancer—Patients—Canada—
Biography. 3. Runners (Sports)—Canada—Biography.
4. Readers for new literates. I. Title. II. Series: Barber, Terry,
1950– . Maple leaf series.

PE1126.N43B3665 2011   428.6'2   C2011–904433–1

Printed in Canada

Contents

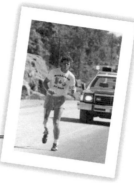

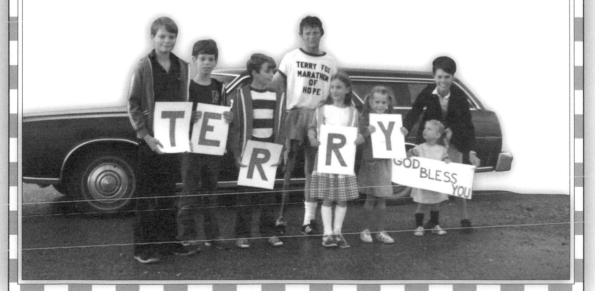

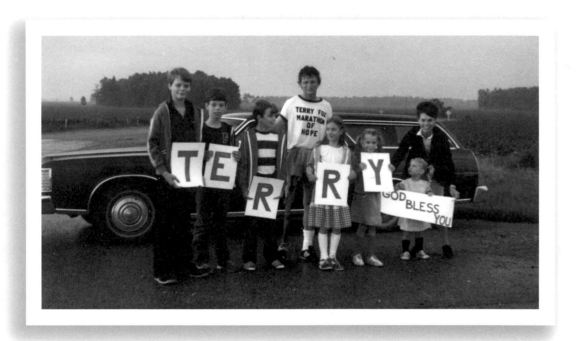

Terry meets a mother and her children.

Memories

The children stand by the road. The sun rises. The rain stops. "Terry's coming!" Dad says. The children hold up their signs. Terry stops to talk with them. Mom and the children stand with Terry. Dad takes a picture.

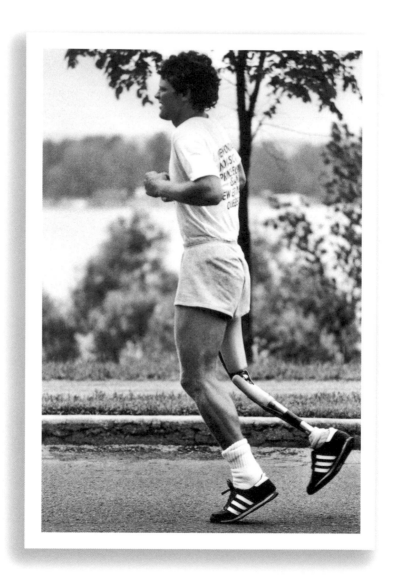

Terry runs down the highway.

Memories

Terry says goodbye. Terry runs west, towards home. The children watch. They are so happy Terry stopped. Terry will run 42 km (26 miles) today. Terry runs a **marathon** most days. The day is warm. What a change from the start of his Marathon of Hope.

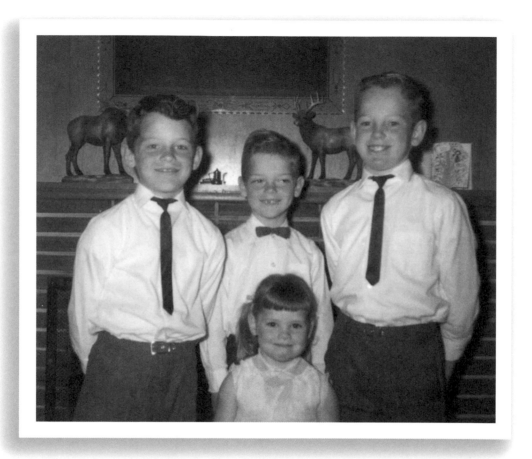

Terry, Darrell, Fred, and Judith Fox (left to right)

The Fox Family

Terry Fox is born in 1958. His father works for the CN Railway. His mother stays home to raise the children. Terry has two brothers and a sister. Terry's family moves to British Columbia in 1966. Terry enjoys a great family life.

Terry Fox is born on July 28 in Winnipeg.

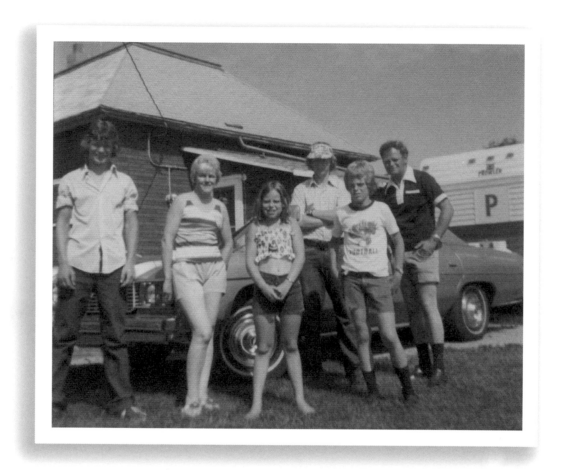

Fox family vacation

The Fox Family

The Fox family is very close. The children learn manners. The children learn respect for others. They learn to stay out of trouble. The children love sports. They have something else in common. They can be stubborn.

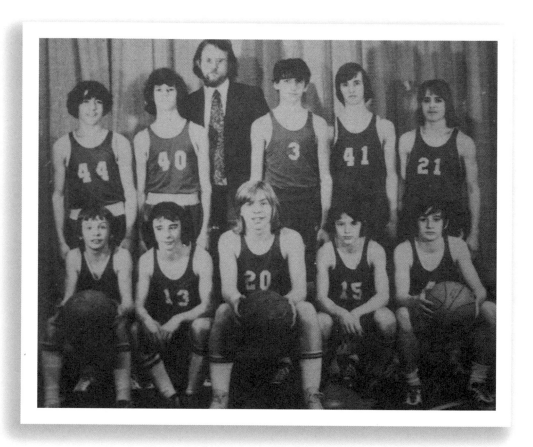

Grade 9 basketball team
Terry (#15), Doug (#13)

The Athlete

Terry loves to play basketball. He plays on the Grade 8 basketball team. Terry is the worst player. His best friend, Doug, plays the sport well.

Terry is stubborn. And he has self-discipline. Terry works hard to become a better player.

Terry also loves to play soccer, rugby, and baseball.

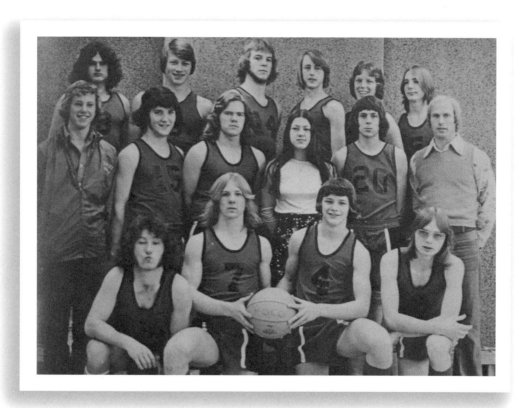

High school basketball team
Terry (#4)

The Athlete

Terry starts high school. He practises basketball every spare moment. Terry becomes the team's best player. Terry becomes captain of the team. Terry never gives up. Terry likes to finish what he starts.

In Grade 12, Terry and Doug share the Athlete of the Year award.

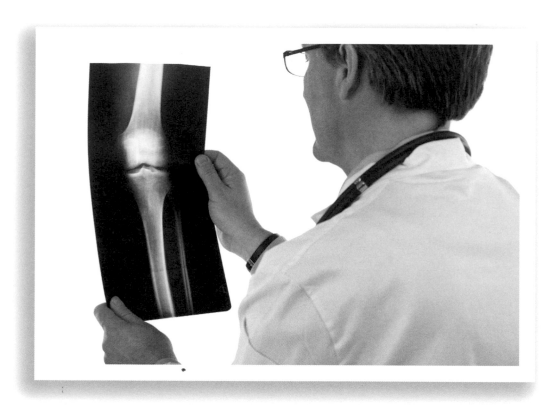

A doctor looks at a knee X-ray.

The Shocking News

Terry turns 18. He is in a car crash. He walks away with a sore knee. The pain does not go away. Terry goes to see his doctor. Terry learns he has bone cancer. Doctors must remove his right leg just above his knee.

Terry has 16 months of **chemotherapy**.

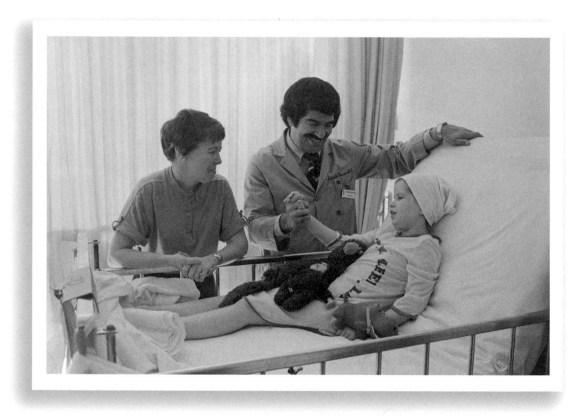

An 8-year-old child with cancer.
1980

The Dream

Terry meets other cancer patients. Some are brave. Some have lost hope. Terry has a dream. He wants to raise money for cancer research. Terry reads about an **amputee** who runs marathons. This man **inspires** Terry. Terry plans his Marathon of Hope.

Terry believes cancer research will help save people's lives.

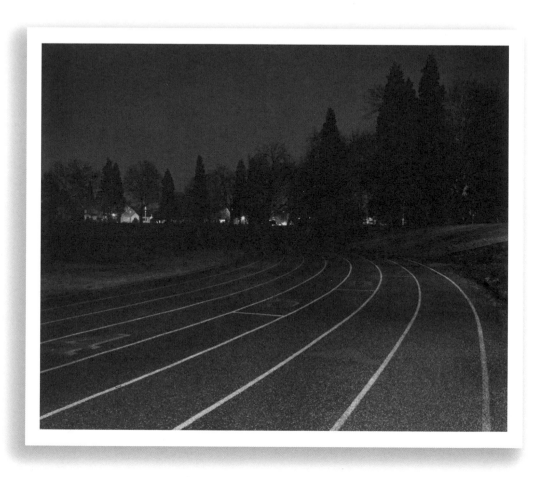

At first, Terry trains at night.

The Dream

Terry trains for the Marathon of Hope. At first, Terry runs in the dark. He is shy about his **artificial** leg. After a while, Terry runs in the day. Terry trains for more than a year. Then, he shares his dream with his family.

Terry runs over 5,000 km (3,100 miles) during his training.

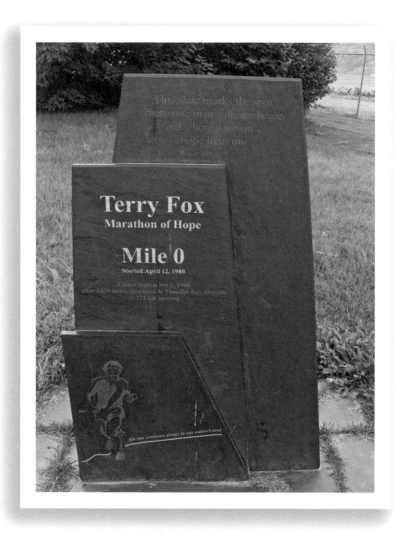

Terry begins his run in St. John's, Newfoundland.
April 12, 1980

The Dream

Terry plans to run across Canada. He
wants to raise money to fight cancer.
He hopes to raise $1 million. Terry
also wants to raise hope in cancer
victims. Terry wants to show how one
person can make a difference.

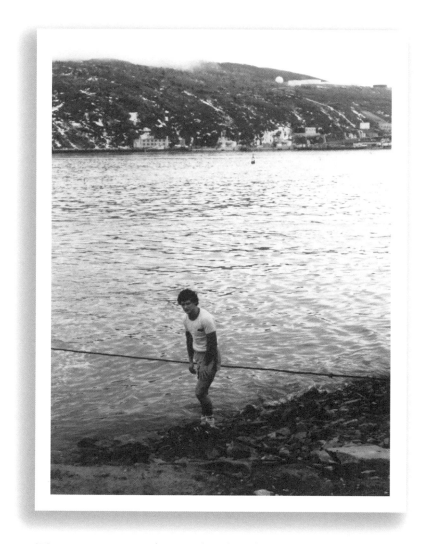

Terry gets ready to dip his leg into the ocean.

The Marathon
of Hope

The Marathon of Hope begins on
April 12, 1980. Winter still hangs in
the air. Terry dips his artificial leg in
the Atlantic Ocean. He puts water
from the ocean into a jug. Terry plans
to pour this water into the Pacific
Ocean.

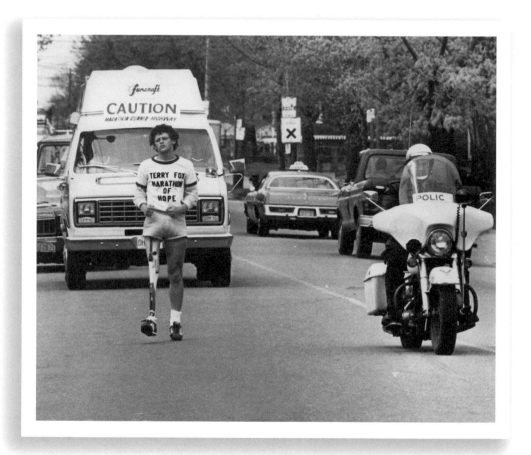

Doug follows Terry in the van
for the entire Marathon.

The Marathon of Hope

Terry needs a driver and a helper.
Terry asks his friend, Doug, to help
him. Doug helps in many ways.
Each day, Terry runs mile after mile.
Doug follows Terry in the van. Doug
hands Terry water when he needs a
drink.

The van
is Doug and
Terry's home.

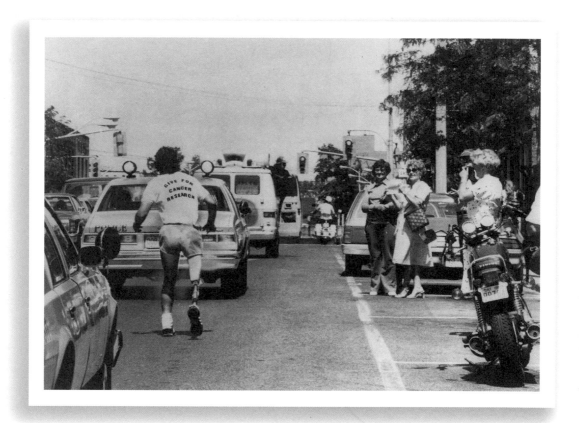

People cheer for Terry.

The Marathon of Hope

Terry runs across the **Atlantic provinces.** He runs across Quebec. The Marathon of Hope builds. As he runs, Terry raises money. The run is hard. Terry won't give up. He keeps running. Crowds of people cheer him on.

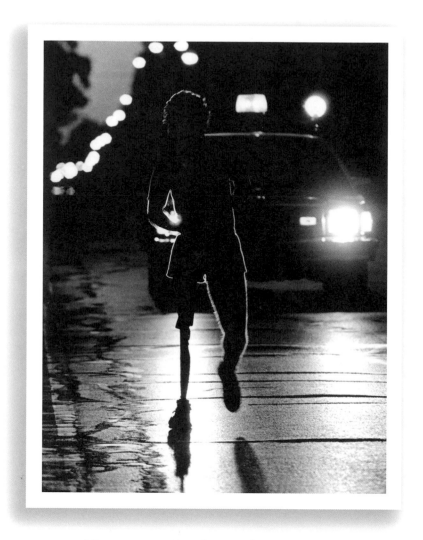

Terry runs in the early morning.
July 13, 1980

The Daily Grind

Imagine being Terry. You do not sleep well. The alarm rings at 4:30 a.m. You must run in the rain. Every step hurts. Your stump bleeds. You must run 26 miles. And you do the same thing the next day. And the next.

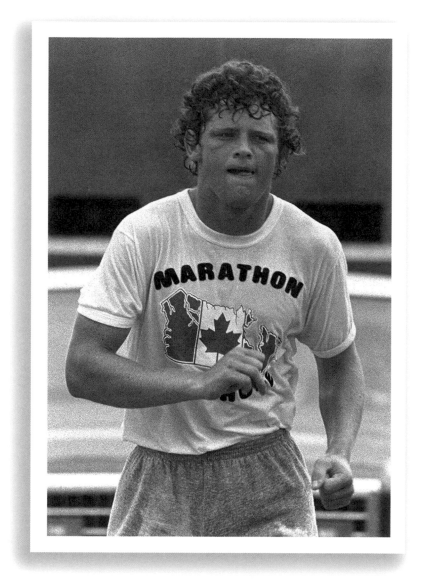

Terry is tired, but he keeps running.

The Daily Grind

Every day is a **grind.** Terry's body wears down. Terry and Doug spend day after day together. They often sleep in the van. The van smells like sweat. The toilet stinks. Terry and Doug argue. Both are under stress.

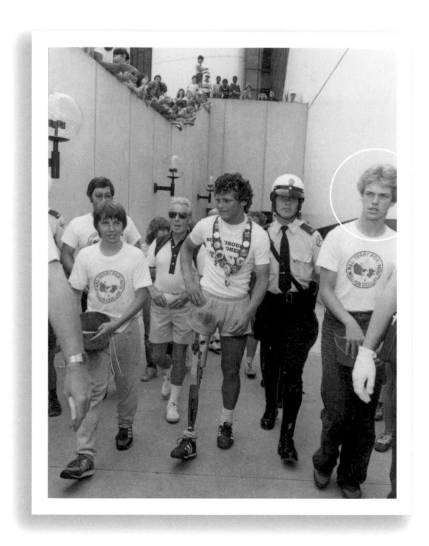

Darrell joins the Marathon of Hope.

The Daily Grind

Terry's parents worry. They want
Terry and Doug to stay best friends.
The family decides that Terry's brother
can help. Darrell joins the Marathon
of Hope. Terry is happy to have his
younger brother with him.

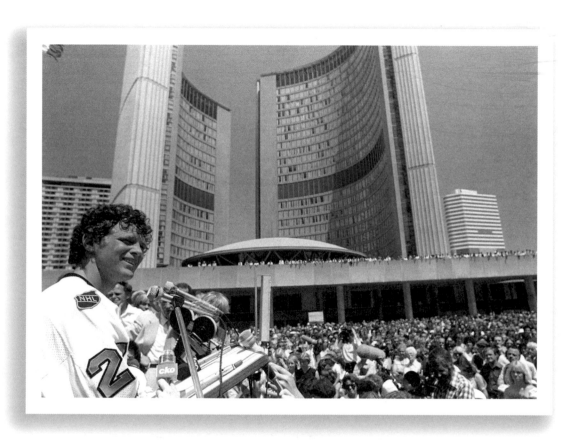

Terry gives a speech in Toronto.

July 11, 1980

The Canadian Hero

In Ontario, Terry's run kicks into high gear. The media focus on Terry's run. Terry is on radio. Terry is on TV. Terry speaks to big groups of people. Canadians want to help. Terry's Marathon of Hope raises more money.

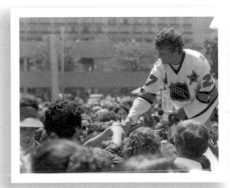

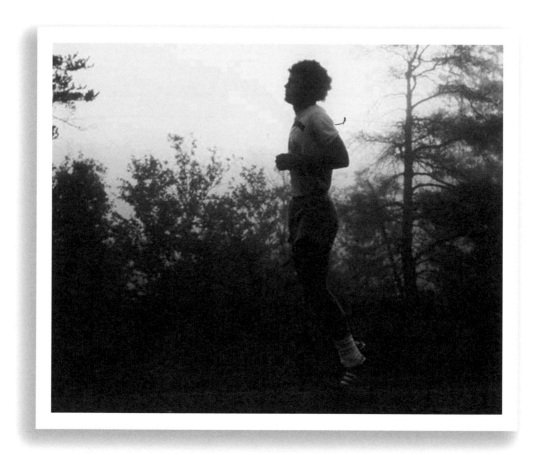

Terry is thin, but he keeps running.

The Canadian Hero

Terry looks less strong. He has lost weight. He coughs a lot. Terry says his run has "got to keep going." Maybe Terry knows he cannot finish his run. He keeps going. He does not lose sight of his goal.

Terry says, "I believe in miracles."

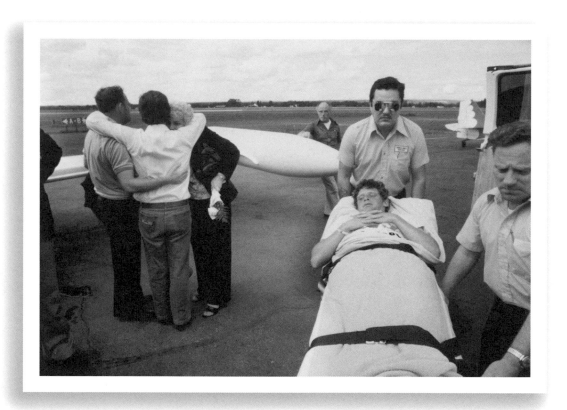

Terry goes home on a plane.

The Canadian Hero

Terry runs for 143 days. He runs 5,373 km (3,339 miles). Then his run ends. The date is September 1, 1980. Terry's cancer has spread to his lungs. He returns home to his family. Terry dies on June 28, 1981. He is only 22 years old.

The Marathon of Hope raises $24.1 million.

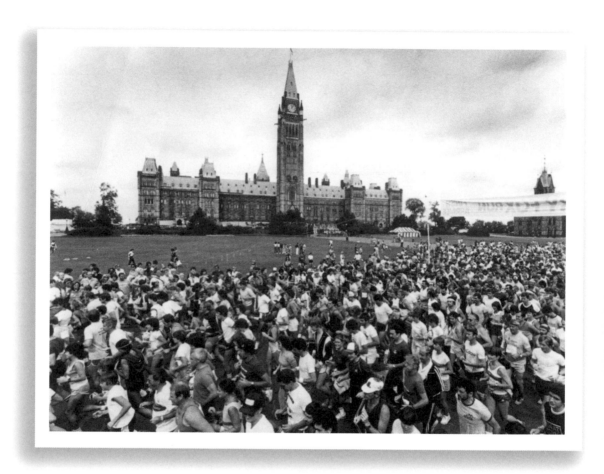

Terry Fox Run
Ottawa, Ontario, 1983

The Terry Fox Run

Terry's dream lives on. The first Terry Fox Run is held in 1981. Today, people around the world enjoy the Terry Fox Run. The run raises money for cancer research. People run to find a **cure** for cancer.

Most people have lost or will lose someone they love to cancer.

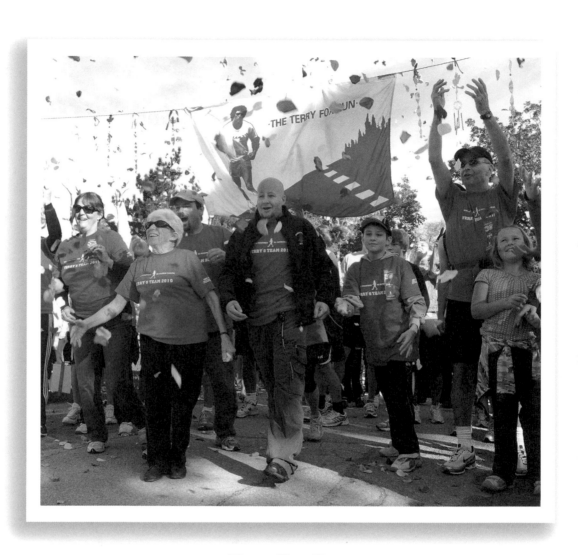

Terry Fox Run
Barrie, Ontario, 2010

The Terry Fox Run

The Fox family still has the water Terry took from the Atlantic Ocean. Terry never got to pour the water into the Pacific Ocean. Terry could not complete his run. But Terry's spirit lives on. Now we run for him.

Terry is the youngest person to get the Order of Canada.

Glossary

amputee: a person who has lost part or all of an arm or leg.

artificial: made by humans.

Atlantic provinces: New Brunswick, Newfoundland, Nova Scotia and Prince Edward Island.

chemotherapy: the treatment of cancer with anti-cancer drugs.

cure: recovery from a disease.

grind: steady, hard work.

inspire: to motivate.

marathon: a long-distance running race that is 42 km (26 miles).

Talking About the Book

What did you learn about Terry Fox?

What words would you use to describe Terry?

Did Terry achieve his dream?

Terry believed in miracles and hope.
Do you believe in the power of hope?
Discuss.

How did Terry make the world
a better place?

Picture Credits